Clinical practice handbook for
Safe abortion

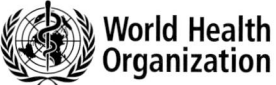

Acknowledgements: WHO is very grateful for the technical contributions of both external experts and past and present WHO staff who informed the development of this document.

WHO Library Cataloguing-in-Publication Data

Clinical practice handbook for safe abortion.

1.Abortion, Induced – methods. 2.Abortion, Induced – standards. 3.Practice guideline. I.World Health Organization.

ISBN 978 92 4 154871 7   (NLM classification: WQ 440)

© **World Health Organization 2014**

All rights reserved. Publications of the World Health Organization are available on the WHO website (www.who.int) or can be purchased from WHO Press, World Health Organization, 20 Avenue Appia, 1211 Geneva 27, Switzerland (tel.: +41 22 791 3264; fax: +41 22 791 4857; e-mail: bookorders@who.int).

Requests for permission to reproduce or translate WHO publications – whether for sale or for non-commercial distribution – should be addressed to WHO Press through the WHO website (www.who.int/about/licensing/copyright_form/en/index.html).

The designations employed and the presentation of the material in this publication do not imply the expression of any opinion whatsoever on the part of the World Health Organization concerning the legal status of any country, territory, city or area or of its authorities, or concerning the delimitation of its frontiers or boundaries. Dotted lines on maps represent approximate border lines for which there may not yet be full agreement.

The mention of specific companies or of certain manufacturers' products does not imply that they are endorsed or recommended by the World Health Organization in preference to others of a similar nature that are not mentioned. Errors and omissions excepted, the names of proprietary products are distinguished by initial capital letters.

All reasonable precautions have been taken by the World Health Organization to verify the information contained in this publication. However, the published material is being distributed without warranty of any kind, either expressed or implied. The responsibility for the interpretation and use of the material lies with the reader. In no event shall the World Health Organization be liable for damages arising from its use.

Printed in Malta

Design and layout by ACW, London

Abbreviations

AIDS	acquired immunodeficiency syndrome
D&E	dilatation and evacuation
EVA	electric vacuum aspiration
Hb	haemoglobin
hCG	human chorionic gonadotrophin
HIV	human immunodeficiency virus
ICD	*International statistical classification of diseases*
IM	intramuscular
IUD	intrauterine device
IV	intravenous
LMP	last menstrual period
MVA	manual vacuum aspiration
NSAID	non-steroidal anti-inflammatory drug
POC	products of conception
Rh	Rhesus (blood group)
STI	sexually transmitted infection
VA	vacuum aspiration
WHO	World Health Organization

Definitions

Duration or gestational age of pregnancy

The number of days or weeks since the first day of the woman's last normal menstrual period (LMP) in women with regular cycles (for women with irregular cycles, the gestational age may need to be determined by physical or ultrasound examination). The first trimester is generally considered to consist of the first 12 or, by some experts, as the first 14 weeks of pregnancy. Throughout this document, gestational age is defined in both weeks and days, reflecting its definition in the *International statistical classification of diseases* (ICD)[*].

Medical methods of abortion (medical abortion)

Use of pharmacological drugs to terminate pregnancy. Sometimes the terms "non-surgical abortion" or "medication abortion" are also used.

Osmotic dilators

Short, thin rods made of seaweed (laminaria) or synthetic material. After placement in the cervical os, the dilators absorb moisture and expand, gradually dilating the cervix.

Surgical methods of abortion (surgical abortion)

Use of transcervical procedures for terminating pregnancy, including vacuum aspiration, and dilatation and evacuation (D&E).

---

[*] International statistical classification of diseases and health related problems, 10th revision – ICD-10, Vol. 2, 2008 edition. Geneva: World Health Organization; 2009.

Purpose of the handbook

The *Clinical practice handbook for safe abortion is* intended to facilitate the practical application of the clinical recommendations from the second edition of *Safe abortion: technical and policy guidance for health systems* (World Health Organization [WHO] 2012). While legal, regulatory, policy and service-delivery contexts may vary from country to country, the recommendations and best practices described in both of these documents aim to enable evidence-based decision-making with respect to safe abortion.

This handbook is oriented to providers who already have the requisite skills and training necessary to provide safe abortion and/or treat complications of unsafe abortion. It is neither a substitute for formal training, nor a training manual.

We hope this handbook will be useful to a range of providers in different settings and in varying legal and health service contexts.

Guiding principles

Providers should be aware of local laws and reporting requirements. Within the framework of national laws, all norms, standards, and clinical practice related to abortion should promote and protect:

- women's and adolescents' health and their human rights;
- informed and voluntary decision-making;
- autonomy in decision-making;
- non-discrimination;
- confidentiality and privacy.

Some practical examples of how providers can apply these principles include:

- treating all women equally regardless of age, ethnicity, socioeconomic or marital status, etc., in a prompt and timely fashion;
- ensuring that abortion care is delivered in a manner that respects all women as decision-makers;
- providing complete, accurate and easy to understand information;
- respecting the dignity of the woman, guaranteeing her privacy and confidentiality;
- being sensitive to the needs and perspectives of the woman;
- protecting medical information against unauthorized disclosures;
- being aware of situations in which a woman may be coerced into having an abortion against her will (e.g. based on her health status, such as living with HIV);
- when dealing with adolescents, encouraging parents' engagement through support, information and education. Do not insist on parents' authorization, unless it is a legal requirement.

Contents

1 PRE-ABORTION
1.1	Information, counselling and decision-making	10
1.2	Medical history	14
1.3	Physical examination	16
1.4	Laboratory and other investigations (if necessary and available)	18
1.5	Discussing contraceptive options	19

2 ABORTION
2.1	Summary of methods: medical and surgical abortion	22
2.2	Infection prevention and control	24
2.3	Pain management	25
2.4	Medical abortion	28
2.5	Medical abortion: ≤12 weeks (or ≤84 days) of pregnancy	29
2.6	Medical abortion: >12 weeks (or >84 days) of pregnancy	34
2.7	Surgical abortion: cervical preparation	37
2.8	Drugs, supplies and equipment for surgical abortion	40
2.9	Surgical abortion: ≤12–14 weeks of pregnancy	42
2.10	Surgical abortion: >12–14 weeks of pregnancy	49

3 POST-ABORTION
3.1	Prior to discharge from the health-care facility	56
3.2	Additional follow-up with a health-care provider	57
3.3	Post-abortion contraception	58
3.4	Assessing and managing abortion complications	61

SECTION 1

PRE-ABORTION

- Information, counselling and decision-making
- Medical history
- Physical examination
- Laboratory and other investigations (if necessary and available)
- Discussing contraceptive options

OBJECTIVES

- Provide information and offer counselling in a way that a woman can understand, to allow her to make her own decisions about whether to have an abortion, and, if so, what method to choose.
- Confirm pregnancy status and determine intrauterine location and gestational duration.
- Evaluate for any medical conditions that require management or may influence the choice of abortion procedure.
- Provide an opportunity to discuss future use of contraception.

1.1 Information, counselling and decision-making

Provide information

Information is a necessary component of any medical care and should always be provided to women considering abortion. At a minimum, this should include,
- the abortion methods and pain management options that she may choose from;
- what will be done before, during and after the procedure, including any tests that may be performed;
- what she is likely to experience (e.g. pain and bleeding) and how long the process is likely to take;
- how to recognize potential complications, and how and where to seek help, if required;
- when she will be able to resume her normal activities, including sexual intercourse;
- follow-up care, including future prevention of unintended pregnancy;
- any legal or reporting requirements.

Most women who have a safe abortion will not suffer any long-term effects (e.g. adverse outcomes in subsequent pregnancies, negative psychological consequences, breast cancer) on their general or reproductive health as a consequence of the abortion.

Offer counselling

Counselling is a focused, interactive process through which one voluntarily receives support, additional information and guidance from a trained person, in an environment that is conducive to openly sharing thoughts, feelings and perceptions. When providing counselling, remember to:
- communicate information in simple language;
- maintain privacy;
- support and ensure adequate response to the questions and needs of the woman;
- avoid imposing personal values and beliefs.

Decision-making

If the woman chooses to have an abortion and a choice of abortion methods is available, she should be allowed to choose among available methods that are appropriate, based on the duration of pregnancy and her medical condition. Adequate and scientifically accurate information about potential risk factors and the advantages and disadvantages of each available method is key to helping her make a choice.

Recommended methods of abortion
by pregnancy duration

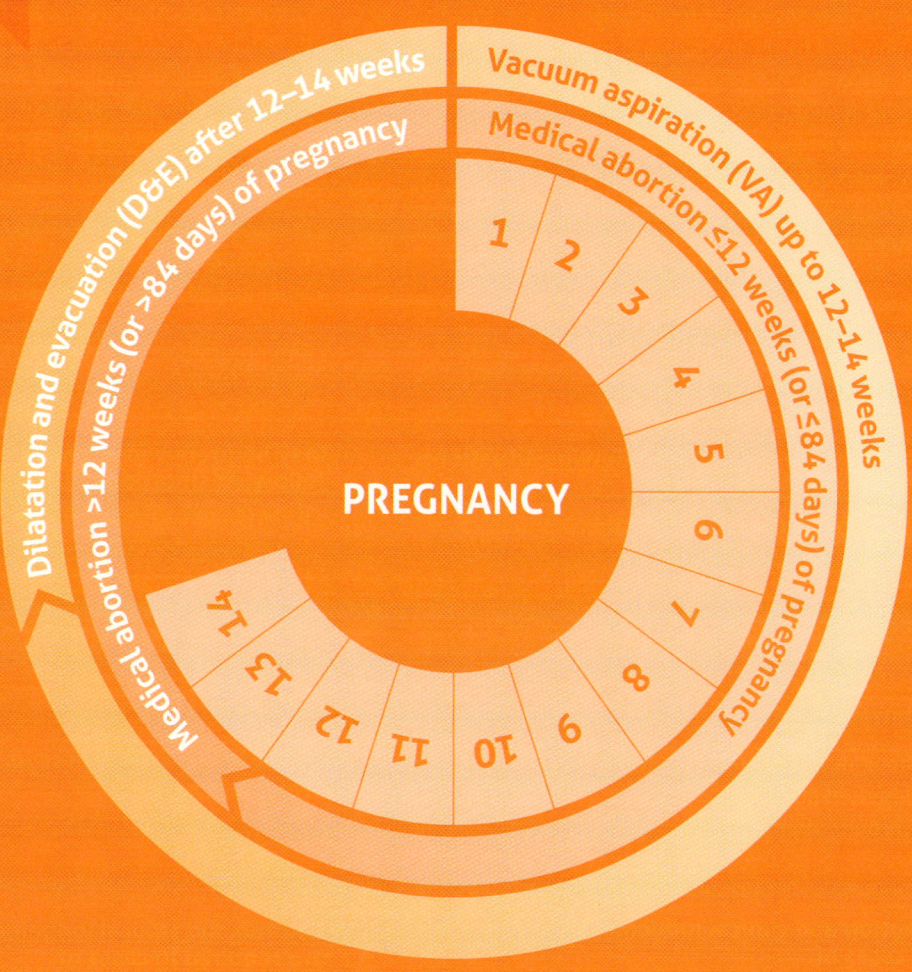

Characteristics of abortion procedures

≤12–14 WEEKS

Medical abortion	**Vacuum aspiration**
▪ Avoids surgery ▪ Mimics the process of miscarriage ▪ Controlled by the woman and may take place at home (< 9 weeks) ▪ Takes time (hours to days) to complete abortion, and the timing may not be predictable ▪ Women experience bleeding and cramping, and potentially some other side-effects (nausea, vomiting) ▪ May require more clinic visits than VA	▪ Quick procedure ▪ Complete abortion easily verified by evaluation of aspirated POC ▪ Takes place in a health-care facility ▪ Sterilization or placement of an intrauterine device (IUD) may be performed at the same time as the procedure ▪ Requires instrumentation of the uterus ▪ Small risk of uterine or cervical injury ▪ Timing of abortion controlled by the facility and provider
May be preferred in the following situations: ▪ For severely obese women ▪ Presence of uterine malformations or fibroids, or previous cervical surgery ▪ If the woman wants to avoid surgical intervention ▪ If a pelvic exam is not feasible or unwanted	**May be preferred in the following situations:** ▪ If there are contraindications to medical abortion ▪ If there are constraints for the timing of the abortion

Contraindications

▪ Previous allergic reaction to one of the drugs involved ▪ Inherited porphyria ▪ Chronic adrenal failure ▪ Known or suspected ectopic pregnancy (neither misoprostol nor mifepristone will treat ectopic pregnancy)	▪ There are no known absolute contraindications
Caution and clinical judgement are required in cases of: ▪ Long-term corticosteroid therapy (including those with severe uncontrolled asthma) ▪ Haemorrhagic disorder ▪ Severe anaemia ▪ Pre-existing heart disease or cardiovascular risk factors ▪ IUD in place (remove before beginning the regimen)	**Caution and clinical judgement are required in cases of:** ▪ IUD in place (remove before beginning the procedure)

>12–14 WEEKS

Medical abortion	Dilatation and evacuation (D&E)
- Avoids surgery - Mimics the process of miscarriage - Takes place in a health-care facility - Takes time (hours to days) to complete abortion, and the timing may not be predictable - Women experience bleeding and cramping, and potentially some other side-effects (nausea, vomiting) - Women remain in the facility until expulsion of the pregnancy is complete - Women with a uterine scar have a very low risk (0.28%) of uterine rupture during medical abortion between 12 and 24 weeks	- Quick procedure - Complete abortion easily verified by evaluation of aspirated POC - Takes place in a health-care facility - Sterilization or placement of an IUD may be performed at the same time as the procedure - Requires cervical preparation in advance of procedure - Requires instrumentation of the uterus - Small risk of uterine or cervical injury - Timing of abortion controlled by the facility and provider
May be preferred in the following situations: - For severely obese women - The presence of uterine malformations or fibroids, or previous cervical surgery - If the woman wants to avoid surgical intervention - If skilled, experienced providers are not available to provide D&E	**May be preferred in the following situations:** - If there are contraindications to medical abortion - If there are time constraints for the abortion

Contraindications

- Previous allergic reaction to one of the drugs involved - Inherited porphyria - Chronic adrenal failure - Known or suspected ectopic pregnancy (neither misoprostol nor mifepristone will treat ectopic pregnancy)	- There are no known absolute contraindications for the use of D&E
Caution and clinical judgement are required in cases of: - Long-term corticosteroid therapy (including those with severe uncontrolled asthma) - Haemorrhagic disorder - Severe anaemia - Pre-existing heart disease or cardiovascular risk factors - IUD in place (remove before beginning the regimen)	**Caution and clinical judgement are required in cases of:** - IUD in place (remove before beginning the regimen)

1.2 Medical history

In addition to estimating the duration of pregnancy, clinical history-taking should serve to identify contraindications to medical or surgical abortion methods and to identify risk factors for complications.

ELEMENTS OF MEDICAL HISTORY	
Personal data	• Name, age and contact information, if possible.
Reason for seeking medical care	• Circumstances of the pregnancy, including pregnancy symptoms or possible complications, such as vaginal bleeding.
Obstetric history	• Details of previous pregnancies and their outcomes, including: ectopic pregnancy, prior miscarriage or abortion, fetal deaths, live births and mode of delivery.

Gynaecologic history	• First date of LMP and whether the last period was normal.
	• Menstrual cycle pattern.
	• Gynaecologic issues, including previous gynaecologic surgery, history of female genital mutilation, or other known physical abnormalities or conditions.
	• Contraceptive history:
	  ▫ current contraceptive use;
	  ▫ contraceptive methods used in the past and experience (positive or negative) with these methods.

Sexual history	• Current partner(s) and whether current partner(s) may have other partner(s). • History or symptoms of any sexually transmitted infections (STIs) including human immunodeficiency virus/acquired immunodeficiency syndrome (HIV/AIDS).

ELEMENTS OF MEDICAL HISTORY	
Surgical/ medical history	- Chronic diseases, such as hypertension, seizure disorder, blood-clotting disorders, liver disease, heart disease, diabetes, sickle-cell anaemia, asthma, significant psychiatric disease. - Details of past hospitalizations. - Details of past surgical operations.
Medications and allergies	- Daily medications. - Use of recent medications or herbal remedies, including any medications and the details of their use (dose, route, timing) if self-abortion was attempted. - Allergy to medications.
Social history	- Marital or partner status. - Family environment. - Violence or coercion by partner or family members. - Other social issues that could impact her care. - History and current use of alcohol and illicit drugs. Note: Health-care providers may encounter women with complicated social situations in the context of providing medical services. Facilitating referral to services to meet women's needs is an important aspect of quality abortion care; however, social history (e.g. marital status) should not be used to create additional barriers to care.

1.3 Physical examination

ELEMENTS OF PHYSICAL EXAMINATION	
General health assessment	- General appearance. - Vital signs. - Signs of weakness, lethargy, anaemia or malnourishment. - Signs or marks of physical violence. - General physical examination (as indicated).
Abdominal examination	- Palpate for the uterus, noting the size and whether tenderness is present. - Note any other abdominal masses. - Note any abdominal scars from previous surgery.

Pelvic examination (speculum and bimanual examination)	- Explain what she can expect during the pelvic examination.
	- Examine the external genitalia for abnormalities or signs of disease or infection.
	
	Speculum examination
	- Inspect the cervix and vaginal canal:
	  - look for abnormalities or foreign bodies;
	  - look for signs of infection, such as pus or other discharge from the cervical os; if pus or other discharge is present, sample for culture, if possible, and administer antibiotics before aspiration;
	  - cervical cytology may be performed at this point, if indicated and available.
	
	Bimanual examination
	- Note the size, shape, position and mobility of the uterus.
	- Assess for adnexal masses.
	- Assess for tenderness of the uterus on palpation or with motion of the cervix, and/or tenderness of the rectovaginal space (cul-de-sac), which may indicate infection.
	- Confirm pregnancy status and pregnancy duration.

Pregnancy dating
by physical examination*

After 4 weeks' gestation, the uterus increases in size by approximately 1 cm per week.

After 15–16 weeks' gestation, the uterus reaches the midpoint between the symphysis pubis and the umbilicus.

| 2 | 4 | 8 | 12 | 16 | 20 | 30 | 40 |

Uterine size (in weeks)

After 12 weeks' gestation, the uterus rises out of the pelvis.

At 20 weeks' gestation, the uterus reaches the umbilicus.

After 20 weeks' gestation, fundal height in centimetres measured from the symphysis pubis approximates the weeks of gestation.

Limitations to dating
by uterine size on physical examination

- Uterine malformations/fibroids.
- Multiple gestation.
- Marked uterine retroversion.
- Obesity.
- Molar pregnancy.

Key considerations

A uterus that is smaller than expected may indicate:

- the woman is not pregnant;
- inaccurate menstrual dating;
- ectopic pregnancy or abnormal intrauterine pregnancy, e.g. spontaneous or missed abortion.

A uterus that is larger than expected may indicate:

- inaccurate menstrual dating;
- multiple gestation;
- uterine abnormalities, such as fibroids;
- molar pregnancy.

*Goodman S, Wolfe M and the TEACH Trainers Collaborative Working Group. Early abortion training workbook, 3rd ed. San Francisco: UCSF Bixby Center for Reproductive Health Research & Policy; 2007.

1.4 Laboratory and other investigations
(if necessary and available)

The following tests, when available, may be performed on the basis of individual risk factors, findings on physical examination, and available resources:

- pregnancy test if pregnancy is unconfirmed;
- haemoglobin (Hb) or haematocrit for suspected anaemia;
- Rhesus (Rh)-testing, where Rh-immunoglobulin is available for Rh-negative women;
- HIV testing/counselling;
- STI screening (usually performed during the pelvic examination);
- cervical cancer screening (performed during the pelvic examination);
- other laboratory tests as indicated by medical history (kidney or liver function tests, etc.);
- diagnostic ultrasound, if indicated, to confirm pregnancy dating or the location of the pregnancy.

IMPORTANT

Routine laboratory testing is not a prerequisite for abortion services.

Discussing contraceptive options 1.5

Immediate initiation of contraception following abortion has been shown to both improve adherence and reduce the risk of unintended pregnancy.

Provide information and offer counselling

- Inform all women that ovulation can return within 2 weeks following abortion, putting them at risk of pregnancy unless an effective contraceptive method is used.
- If the woman is interested in contraception, she requires accurate information to assist her in choosing the most appropriate contraceptive method to meet her needs.
- Understand that some women prefer to discuss options for contraception after the abortion is completed.
- If a woman is seeking an abortion following what she considers to be a contraceptive failure, discuss whether the method may have been used incorrectly and how to use it correctly, or whether it may be appropriate for her to change to a different method.
- Ultimately, the final decision about whether to use contraception, and identification of a method to use, is the woman's alone.

IMPORTANT

A woman's acceptance of a contraceptive method must never be a precondition for providing her an abortion.

SECTION 2

ABORTION

- Summary of methods: medical and surgical abortion
- Infection prevention and control
- Pain management
- Medical abortion:
  - ≤12 weeks (or ≤84 days) of pregnancy
  - >12 weeks (or >84 days) of pregnancy
- Surgical abortion:
  - Cervical preparation
  - Drugs, supplies and equipment
  - ≤12–14 weeks of pregnancy
  - >12–14 weeks of pregnancy

2.1 Summary of methods: medical and surgical abortion

Medical abortion

UP TO 9 WEEKS (63 DAYS)	9–12 WEEKS (63–84 DAYS)

MIFEPRISTONE & MISOPROSTOL

- Mifepristone 200 mg
- Oral
- Single dose

UP TO 9 WEEKS (63 DAYS)	9–12 WEEKS (63–84 DAYS)
- Misoprostol 800 μg - Vaginal, buccal or sublingual - Single dose OR *If no more than 7 weeks (49 days)* - Misoprostol 400 μg - Oral - Single dose - Use **24–48 hours** after taking mifepristone	- Misoprostol 800 μg, then 400 μg - Vaginal, then vaginal or sublingual - Every 3 hours up to 5 doses - Start **36–48 hours** after taking mifepristone

MISOPROSTOL ALONE

- Misoprostol 800 μg
- Vaginal or sublingual
- Every **3-12 hours** up to 3 doses

Surgical abortion

≤12–14 WEEKS

Vacuum aspiration

Methods of vacuum aspiration include:
- manual vacuum aspiration (MVA)
- electric vacuum aspiration (EVA)

>12 WEEKS (84 DAYS)

- Misoprostol 800 μg, then 400 μg
- Vaginal, then vaginal or sublingual

OR

- Misoprostol 400 μg, then 400 μg
- Oral, then vaginal or sublingual
- Every 3 hours up to 5 doses
- Start use **36–48 hours** after taking mifepristone

- Misoprostol 400 μg
- Vaginal or sublingual
- Every **3 hours** up to 5 doses

For pregnancies beyond 24 weeks, the dose of misoprostol should be reduced, owing to the greater sensitivity of the uterus to prostaglandins, but the lack of clinical studies precludes specific dosing recommendations.

>12–14 WEEKS

Dilatation and evacuation (D&E)
D&E is the surgical method for abortion >12–14 weeks of pregnancy.

2.2 Infection prevention and control

Since abortion procedures and care involve contact with blood and other body fluids, all clinical and support staff that provide these services should understand and apply standard precautions for infection prevention and control, for both their own protection and that of their patients.

Standard precautions, also called universal precautions:

- should be applied in all situations where health-care workers anticipate contact with: blood; any body fluid other than perspiration; non-intact skin; and mucous membranes;
- should always be followed, regardless of a person's presumed infection status or diagnosis;
- minimize or eliminate transmission of disease from patient to health-care worker, health-care worker to patient, or patient to patient.

Standard precautions

- Hand-washing;
    - hand washing with soap and running water should be routine before and after each contact, including after contact with potentially contaminated items, even if gloves are worn;
    - gloves should be worn and replaced between contacts with different clients and between vaginal (or rectal) examinations of the same woman. After completing care of one woman and removing gloves, the health-care provider should always wash their hands, as gloves may have undetected holes in them.
- Wearing barriers such as gowns, gloves, aprons, masks, protective eyewear and footwear:
    - it should be noted that use of auxiliary supplies, such as sterile booties, does not make a significant difference in infection rates, although it increases costs.
- Aseptic technique:
    - prior to any surgical abortion procedure, the woman's cervix should be cleaned with an antiseptic (e.g. betadine).
- Proper handling and disposal of sharp instruments ("sharps") – blades and needles.
- Proper handling and processing of instruments and materials.

Caution: Aspirators, cannulae and adaptors are not safe to handle with bare hands until cleaned.

Pain management 2.3

Almost all women will experience some pain and cramping with abortion. Neglecting this important element needlessly increases a woman's anxiety and discomfort, potentially lengthening the procedure and compromising her care.

- The amount of pain that women experience with uterine evacuation or pregnancy expulsion, and their response to that pain, varies greatly.
- It is necessary to individually assess each woman's pain-management needs.
- Both non-pharmacological and pharmacological methods may be helpful in reducing pain associated with abortion.
- Close attention should be paid to a woman's medical history, allergies and concurrent use of medications that might interact with any available analgesic or anaesthetic agents, to optimize the safe use of all pain medications.

Understanding pain with abortion

- A woman having an abortion may feel anxiety, fear or apprehension.
    - Anxiety can increase sensitivity to pain.
    - A highly anxious woman may not be able to lie still on the procedure table for a surgical abortion, potentially compromising her safety if this is not treated.
- Pain related to both physiological and mechanical cervical dilatation and uterine contractions is common among women undergoing abortion.

IMPORTANT

Offer all women appropriate pain management before medical or surgical abortion.

Pain-management options

	SURGICAL ABORTION	MEDICAL ABORTION
NON-PHARMACOLOGICAL METHODS	<ul><li>Respectful, non-judgmental communication</li><li>Verbal support and reassurance</li><li>Gentle, smooth operative technique</li><li>Advance notice of each step of the procedure (if the woman desires it)</li><li>The presence of a support person who can remain with her during the process (if the woman desires it)</li><li>Encouraging deep, controlled breathing</li><li>Listening to music</li><li>Hot water bottle or heating pad</li></ul>	<ul><li>Respectful, non-judgmental communication</li><li>Verbal support and reassurance</li><li>Thorough explanation of what to expect</li><li>The presence of a support person who can remain with her during the process (if the woman desires it)</li><li>Hot water bottle or heating pad</li></ul>
PHARMACOLOGICAL METHODS	<ul><li>Analgesia (non-steroidal anti-inflammatory drugs [NSAIDs], e.g. ibuprofen 400–800 mg)</li><li>Anxiolytics/sedatives (e.g. diazepam 5–10 mg)</li><li>Local anaesthetic (paracervical block using lidocaine (usually 10–20 mL of 0.5 to 1.0%)</li><li>Conscious sedation or general anaesthesia in some cases, not routinely</li></ul>	<ul><li>Analgesia (NSAIDs, e.g. ibuprofen 400–800 mg)</li><li>Anxiolytics/sedatives (e.g. diazepam 5–10 mg)</li><li>Adjuvant medications may also be provided, if indicated, for side-effects of misoprostol (e.g. loperamide for diarrhoea).</li><li>**>12 weeks' gestation** In addition to NSAIDs, offer at least one or more of the following:<ul><li>oral opioids;</li><li>intramuscular (IM) or intravenous (IV) opioids; epidural anaesthesia.</li></ul></li></ul>

- Paracetamol is not recommended to decrease pain during abortion.
- To ensure that oral medications will be most effective at the time of the procedure, administer them 30–45 minutes before the procedure.

Example of how to administer a paracervical block*

- Inject 1–2 mL of anaesthetic at the cervical site where the tenaculum will be placed (either at 12 o'clock or 6 o'clock, depending on the preference of the provider or the presentation of the cervix).
- Next, stabilize the cervix with the tenaculum at the anaesthetized site.
- Use slight traction to move the cervix and define the transition of smooth cervical epithelium to vaginal tissue, which delineates the placement for additional injections.
- Slowly inject 2–5 mL lidocaine into a depth of 1.5–3 cm at 2–4 points at the cervical/vaginal junction (2 and 10 o'clock, and/or 4 and 8 o'clock).
- Move the needle while injecting OR aspirate before injecting, to avoid intravascular injection.
- The maximum dose of lidocaine in a paracervical block is 4.5 mg/kg/dose or generally 200–300 mg (approximately 20 mL of 1% or 40 mL of 0.5%).

IMPORTANT

General anaesthesia is not routinely recommended for vacuum aspiration or D&E.

Medications used for general anaesthesia are one of the few potentially life-threatening aspects of abortion care. Any facility that offers general anaesthesia must have the specialized equipment and staff to administer it and to handle complications.

When IV pain management, conscious sedation or general anaesthesia is used, a clinician trained (and certified, if legally required) to monitor appropriate respiratory, cardiovascular and neurologic parameters, including the level of consciousness, must be present. The practitioner administering IV pain management must be prepared to provide respiratory support in the event of respiratory suppression.

Following the recommended dose-range limits reduces greatly any risks associated with these medications. If drugs are used that cause sedation and, potentially, respiratory depression, their antagonists must be available, preferably on an emergency cart, along with instructions on treating adverse reaction.

*Maltzer DS, Maltzer MC, Wiebe ER, Halvorson-Boyd G, Boyd C. Pain management. In: Paul M, Lichtenberg ES, Borgatta L, Grimes DA, Stubblefield PG, editors. A clinician's guide to medical and surgical abortion. New York: Churchill Livingstone; 1999:73–90.

2.4 Medical abortion

Clinical considerations

- Medical abortion is a multistep process involving two medications (mifepristone and misoprostol) and/or multiple doses of one medication (misoprostol alone).

- Mifepristone with misoprostol is more effective than misoprostol used alone, and is associated with fewer side-effects.

- Allowing home use of misoprostol following provision of mifepristone at a health care facility can improve the privacy, convenience and acceptability of services, without compromising on safety. Facility-based abortion care should be reserved for the management of medical abortion for pregnancies over nine weeks (63 days) and management of severe abortion complications.

- Women must be able to access advice and emergency care in the event of complications, if necessary.

- Inform the woman that misoprostol might have teratogenic effects if the abortion fails and the woman decides to continue the pregnancy.

    - There is no need to insist on termination of an exposed pregnancy; data are limited and inconclusive regarding teratogenicity. However, because of potential risk, follow-up of a continued pregnancy is important in this situation.

- Mifepristone and misoprostol do not terminate ectopic pregnancy.

    - Absence of bleeding is a possible indication that the pregnancy may be ectopic, but it may also signify that an intrauterine pregnancy did not abort.

    - Even if a pregnancy is ectopic, a woman can experience some bleeding after taking mifepristone and misoprostol because the decidua may respond to the medications.

    - Evaluate the woman for ectopic pregnancy if she reports signs or symptoms of ongoing pregnancy after medical abortion.

Medical abortion: ≤12 weeks (or ≤84 days) of pregnancy

2.5

Treatment regimens for medical abortion ≤12 weeks (or ≤84 days) of pregnancy

	UP TO 9 WEEKS (63 DAYS)	9–12 WEEKS (63–84 DAYS)
MIFEPRISTONE & MISOPROSTOL	• Mifepristone 200 mg • Oral • Single dose	
	• Misoprostol 800 μg • Vaginal, buccal or sublingual • Single dose OR *If no more than 7 weeks (49 days)* • Misoprostol 400 μg • Oral • Single dose • Use **24–48 hours** after taking mifepristone	• Misoprostol 800 μg, then 400 μg • Vaginal, then vaginal or sublingual • Every 3 hours up to 5 doses • Start **36–48 hours** after taking mifepristone
MISOPROSTOL ALONE	• Misoprostol 800 μg • Vaginal or sublingual • Every **3-12 hours** up to 3 doses	

Providing the abortion procedure

☑ Administer the medication to initiate medical abortion

- Mifepristone is always administered orally.
- Misoprostol can be administered by different routes, including oral, vaginal, buccal and sublingual. Side-effects and instructions for use differ (see Characteristics of different routes of misoprostol administration, p.31).
- Antibiotic prophylaxis is not necessary for medical abortion.

☑ Offer supportive care prior to and during pregnancy expulsion

Ensure that all women have access to information and services to support successful completion of the abortion procedure, address common side-effects and manage any complications that may arise.

- Discuss the range of pain and bleeding associated with the abortion process. Explain the possibility of heavy bleeding with clots, passage of the products of conception, and pain that may be significantly stronger than normal menstrual cramps for some women.
- It is essential that the woman knows to seek medical attention for:
  - prolonged or heavy bleeding (soaking more than two large pads per hour for two consecutive hours);
  - fever lasting more than 24 hours;
  - or feeling generally unwell more than 24 hours after misoprostol administration.

Home use of misoprostol: some considerations

- Ensure that the woman understands when and how to use the misoprostol tablets before she goes home.
- Ensure that the woman understands when and how to self-administer pain medication. Other pain-relieving measures should be reviewed with each woman for use as she prefers.
- Ensure that the woman understands how to contact a health-care provider in the event of questions, concerns or complications.

Facility use of misoprostol: some considerations

- Ensure that the woman has access to private toilets while awaiting pregnancy expulsion.

Characteristics of different routes of misoprostol administration

ROUTE	INSTRUCTIONS FOR USE	NOTES
Oral	Pills are swallowed	- Only recommended up to 7 weeks (49 days) and after 12 weeks (84 days) - Side-effects include diarrhoea and nausea, fever and chills
Buccal	Pills are placed between the cheek and gums and swallowed after 30 minutes	- More fever and chills than with the vaginal route
Sublingual	Pills are placed under the tongue and swallowed after 30 minutes	- Increased fever, chills, diarrhoea and vomiting compared to the vaginal route - Fastest onset of action and highest plasma concentration levels
Vaginal	Pills are placed in the vaginal fornices (deepest portions of the vagina) and the woman is instructed to lie down for 30 minutes	- Pill fragments may be visible - Lowest rate of side-effects

Buccal and sublingual routes of misoprostol administration

Buccal

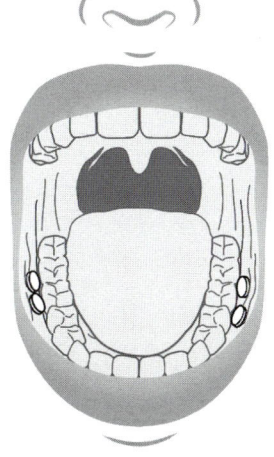

Sublingual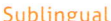

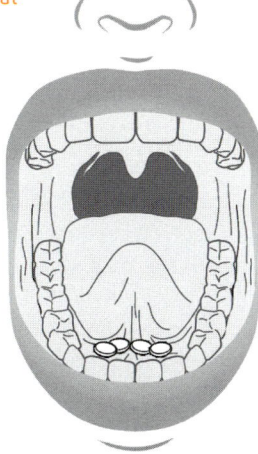

Side-effects and complications and their management

DESCRIPTION	MANAGEMENT
Pain	- Respectful, non-judgmental communication - Verbal support and reassurance - Thorough explanation of what to expect - The presence of a support person who can remain with her during the process (only if she desires it) - Hot water bottle or heating pad - NSAIDs, such as ibuprofen
Bleeding	- Create reasonable expectations about the amount and duration of bleeding - If there is evidence of haemodynamic compromise, start IV fluids - Vacuum aspiration for profuse bleeding - Blood transfusion, if required (rare)
Fever (repeated doses of misoprostol may cause temperature elevation)	- Antipyretic drugs, such as paracetamol - If fever persists for more than 24 hours after misoprostol, further assessment is warranted
Nausea and vomiting	- Self-limiting. Reassure, provide anti-emetics if desired
Diarrhoea	- Self-limiting. Reassure, provide antidiarrhoeal medication if desired - Encourage oral hydration
Pelvic infection	- If infection is suspected, perform physical examination - If infection is confirmed, provide antibiotics and uterine evacuation and hospitalize if necessary

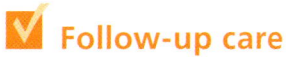 **Follow-up care**

Mifepristone and misoprostol
- There is no medical need for a mandatory routine follow-up. Women should be able to have a follow-up visit if they desire. If a follow-up visit is scheduled, it should be between 7 and 14 days.

Misoprostol alone
- Clinic follow-up to ensure complete abortion is recommended. (This regimen is less effective than the combined regimen.)

Assessing for completed abortion
The use of clinical signs and symptoms with bimanual examination, human chorionic gonadotrophin (hCG) levels or ultrasonography (if available) can confirm abortion completion.

Further evaluation for completed abortion is needed if:
- a woman reports ongoing symptoms of pregnancy and/or has only minimal bleeding after taking the abortifacient medications as directed:
  - ongoing pregnancy should be suspected and further evaluation could include pelvic examination, demonstrating a growing uterus, or an ultrasound scan, demonstrating an ongoing pregnancy;
  - offer vacuum aspiration or repeat administration of misoprostol to complete her abortion;
- a woman reports prolonged or excessive bleeding and cramping, and ongoing intrauterine pregnancy (see above) is not suspected:
  - consider a diagnosis of ectopic pregnancy and manage appropriately;
  - offer repeat misoprostol or vacuum aspiration to complete the abortion;
- a woman reports lighter than expected bleeding or no bleeding, and ongoing intrauterine pregnancy is not suspected:
  - consider a diagnosis of ectopic pregnancy and manage appropriately.

2.6 Medical abortion: >12 weeks (or >84 days) of pregnancy

Clinical considerations

- Administration of misoprostol occurs in the health-care facility.
- Women remain in the facility until expulsion of the pregnancy is complete.
- If the gestational age is beyond 20 weeks, some service providers consider pre-procedure fetal demise.
- Uterine sensitivity to prostaglandins increases with gestational age. The dose of misoprostol therefore decreases as gestational age increases.

Recommendations for medical abortion

>12 WEEKS (OR >84 DAYS)

MIFEPRISTONE & MISOPROSTOL

- Mifepristone 200 mg
- Oral
- Single dose

- Misoprostol 800 µg, then 400 µg
- Vaginal, then vaginal or sublingual

OR

- Misoprostol 400 µg, then 400 µg
- Oral, then vaginal or sublingual
- Every 3 hours up to 5 doses
- Start use **36–48 hours** after taking mifepristone

For pregnancies beyond 24 weeks, the dose of misoprostol should be reduced, owing to the greater sensitivity of the uterus to prostaglandins, but the lack of clinical studies precludes specific dosing recommendations.

MISOPROSTOL ALONE

- Misoprostol 400 µg
- Vaginal or sublingual
- Every **3 hours** up to 5 doses

Providing the abortion procedure

✅ Administer the medication to initiate medical abortion

- Mifepristone is always administered orally.

- Misoprostol may be administered by different routes, including oral, vaginal, buccal and sublingual. Side-effects and instructions for use differ.

- Antibiotic prophylaxis is not necessary for medical abortion.

✅ Ensure prompt administration of repeat misoprostol as necessary and offer supportive care while awaiting pregnancy expulsion

Cramping will often begin before the second dose of misoprostol is administered; however, timing is variable. Starting from the time of the first dose of misoprostol, women should be monitored regularly, particularly in relation to their need for pain management.

The expected time to expulsion and completion of abortion increases with gestational age and with nulliparity.

✅ Fetal/placental expulsion

- If the fetus/products of conception (POC) have not passed after 8–10 hours of receiving misoprostol, perform a vaginal examination, and remove the POC if present in the vagina or cervical os.

- Routine uterine curettage is unwarranted.

    - Use of modern methods of medical abortion (misoprostol with or without mifepristone) results in low rates (<10%) of retained placenta. Uterine evacuation by vacuum aspiration (or curettage, where aspiration is unavailable) to remove the placenta should only be performed in women who have heavy bleeding, fever or a retained placenta beyond 3–4 hours.

✓ Recovery and discharge from facility

- Reassure the woman that the procedure is finished and that she is no longer pregnant.
- Offer to address any emotional needs the woman might have immediately following her abortion.
- Monitor her for any complications and provide management as needed.
- She may leave the facility when she is stable and meets criteria for discharge.
- Ensure that the woman has all necessary information and/or medications prior to leaving the facility.
- Document all outcomes of the treatment, including any adverse events.

NOTE

Fever can be a frequent side-effect of repeated doses of misoprostol; administration of paracetamol or ibuprofen will decrease a woman's discomfort. Fever that persists for hours after the last dose of misoprostol should be evaluated.

Severe pain that persists should be evaluated to rule out uterine rupture, a rare complication.

Surgical abortion: cervical preparation

Cervical preparation before surgical abortion is recommended for all women with pregnancies over 12–14 weeks.

- Though not routinely recommended for pregnancies less than 12 weeks' duration, use of cervical preparation may be considered for all women undergoing surgical abortion. Factors influencing this consideration may include whether the woman is at higher risk for abortion complications, as well as provider experience.

- Adequate cervical preparation decreases the morbidity associated with second-trimester surgical abortion, including the risk of cervical injury, uterine perforation and incomplete abortion.

- Osmotic dilators and pharmacologic agents can be used for cervical preparation.

- Analgesics, such as ibuprofen and/or narcotics, as well as oral anxiolytics as needed, should be administered around the time of cervical preparation and repeated as needed, in advance of the procedure, to maximize their effectiveness.

IMPORTANT

If a woman undergoing cervical preparation starts experiencing heavy vaginal bleeding, she should have the evacuation procedure without delay.

Cervical preparation before surgical abortion

≤12–14 WEEKS

- Placement of laminaria within the cervical canal 6–24 hours prior to the procedure
- Administration of mifepristone

DOSE	ROUTE	TIMING
200 mg	Oral	24–48 hours prior to the procedure

- Administration of misoprostol

DOSE	ROUTE	TIMING
400 µg	Vaginal	3–4 hours prior to the procedure
400 µg	Sublingual	2–3 hours prior to the procedure

NOTE: Vaginal administration provides equally effective dilatation with fewer systemic side-effects than sublingual administration.

>12–14 WEEKS

- Use of misoprostol results in less dilatation than osmotic dilators but has the advantage of being a one-day procedure for most women
- 12–19 weeks' gestation: either misoprostol or osmotic dilators
- Beyond 20 weeks' gestation: osmotic dilators are preferred
- Administration of misoprostol

DOSE	ROUTE	TIMING
400 µg	Vaginal	3–4 hours prior to the procedure

Example of how to insert osmotic dilators

- Place a speculum in the vagina and wipe the cervix with a non-alcoholic antiseptic solution.

- Administer local anaesthesia to the cervical lip, or a full cervical block (see instructions for administering a paracervical block, p.27), then grasp the lip of the cervix with an atraumatic tenaculum.

- Grasp the end of the osmotic device with forceps (ring or packing forceps) and insert it into the endocervical canal such that the tip extends just beyond the internal cervical os. Coating the osmotic dilator with lubricant jelly or with antiseptic solution can ease placement.

- Sequentially place the dilators adjacent to one another within the cervical os, so that they fit snugly in the cervical canal.

Additional considerations for misoprostol and osmotic dilator use for cervical preparation

Osmotic dilators

- Maximum dilatation occurs between 6 and 12 hours after placement. When less than the desired number of osmotic dilators is placed initially, the procedure can be repeated, in 4 hours or the following day, to place additional dilators.

- As there is minimal risk of expulsion after placement of laminaria, women often leave the clinic and return for their procedure at a later scheduled time.

Misoprostol

- Women may experience some bleeding and cramping from the misoprostol.

- Ensure there is a place for women to wait comfortably while the misoprostol is taking effect.

- If the cervix does not dilate easily after one dose of misoprostol, the dose can be repeated.

2.8 Drugs, supplies and equipment for surgical abortion

	CLINICAL ASSESSMENT	VA PROCEDURE AND D&E PROCEDURE
DRUGS AND SUPPLIES	- Clean examination gloves	- Clean water - Detergent or soap - Cervical preparation agent (e.g. misoprostol, mifepristone, osmotic dilators) - Pain medications, such as analgesics and anxiolytics - Gloves - Gown, face protection - Needles (22-gauge spinal for paracervical block and 21-gauge for drug administration) - Syringes (5, 10 and 20 mL) - Lidocaine for paracervical block - Gauze sponges or cotton balls - Antiseptic solution (non-alcohol based) to prepare the cervix - Instrument-soaking solution - Sterilization or high-level disinfection solutions and materials - Silicone for lubricating syringes
EQUIPMENT	- Blood-pressure equipment - Stethoscope	- **Speculum (wide mouth to increase exposure of the cervix and short to avoid pushing the cervix away, or a Sims speculum if an assistant is available)*** - Tenaculum (when available) - **Tapered dilators up to 51 mm or equivalent circumference*** - Stepwise sized cannulae up to 12 or 14 mm - Electric vacuum aspirator (with cannulae up to 12–14 mm) or manual vacuum aspirator (with cannulae up to 12 mm) - **Bierer uterine evacuation forceps (large and small)*** - **Sopher uterine evacuation forceps (small)*** - **Large, postpartum flexible curette*** - Sponge forceps - Stainless steel bowl for prepping solution - Instrument tray - Clear glass dish for tissue inspection - Strainer (metal, glass or gauze)

*Equipment for dilatation and evacuation (D&E) is highlighted in bold font.

RECOVERY	IN CASE OF COMPLICATIONS
- Sanitary napkins or cotton wool - Analgesics - Antibiotics - Information on post-procedure self-care - Post-abortion contraceptive methods and information and/or referral	- Appropriate antagonists to medications used for pain - Uterotonics (oxytocin, misoprostol or ergometrine) - IV line and fluids (saline, sodium lactate, glucose) - Clear referral mechanisms to higher-level facility, when needed
- Blood pressure equipment - Stethoscope	- Oxygen and Ambu bag - On-site access to an ultrasound machine (optional) - Long needle-driver and suture - Scissors - Uterine packing

2.8 Drugs, supplies and equipment for surgical abortion

2.9 Surgical abortion: ≤12–14 weeks of pregnancy

Clinical considerations

There are two types of vacuum aspiration.

- Manual vacuum aspiration (MVA) uses a hand-held aspirator to generate a vacuum. The aspirator is attached to cannulae ranging from 4 to 14 mm in diameter and can be used in multiple settings, including those without electricity.
- Electric vacuum aspiration (EVA) uses an electric pump to generate a vacuum and can accommodate cannulae up to 14–16mm in diameter, with larger-diameter tubing (for cannulae >12 mm).

The abortion procedure is performed similarly, regardless of the type of vacuum used.

Prior to the start of the procedure

- Refer the woman to an appropriate facility, as needed, if conditions are detected that may cause or exacerbate complications.
- Perform cervical preparation, if needed. (Refer to Surgical abortion: cervical preparation Section 2.7, p.37).
- Provide antibiotic prophylaxis to reduce post-procedure infection.
- Confirm that the woman has received her pain medications.
- Ensure that all necessary equipment is gathered and available for use. If using MVA, make sure to check that:
  - the aspirator holds a vacuum before starting the procedure;
  - back-up aspirators are readily available, in case the first aspirator has technical problems.

IMPORTANT

To reduce the risk of post-procedure infection, prophylactic antibiotics initiated preoperatively or perioperatively are recommended: facilities offering surgical abortion should make efforts to secure adequate antibiotic supplies. If antibiotics are not available, however, abortion may still be performed.

Surgical abortion
≤12–14 weeks of pregnancy

1	Ask the woman to empty her bladder
2	Wash hands and put on protective barriers
3	Perform a bimanual examination
4	Place the speculum
5	Perform cervical antiseptic preparation
6	Perform paracervical block (or proceed to Step 7)
7	Dilate the cervix
8	Insert the cannula
9	Aspirate the uterine contents
10	Inspect the tissue
11	Perform any concurrent procedures
12	Recovery and discharge from the facility

> ### THE "NO-TOUCH" TECHNIQUE
>
> Reducing infection after vacuum aspiration is accomplished by using appropriately disinfected or sterilized instruments, administering prophylactic antibiotics, and using the no-touch technique.
>
> The no-touch technique means that the parts of instruments that enter the uterus should not touch objects or surfaces that are not sterile, including the vaginal walls, before being inserted.
>
> Thus, during the aspiration procedure, the provider:
>
> - grasps and touches only the midportion of dilators, avoiding the tips;
> - attaches the cannula to the vacuum source without touching the tip of the cannula;
> - keeps used instruments away from sterile instruments remaining on the tray.
>
> Underlying this technique is the recognition that, even with application of antiseptic solution to the cervix, it is impossible to sterilize the vagina.
>
> Reference: Meckstroth K, Paul M. First trimester aspiration abortion. In: Paul M. Lichtenberg ES, Borgatta L, Grimes DA, Stubblefield PG, Creinin MD, editors. Management of unintended and abnormal pregnancy: comprehensive abortion care. Oxford: Blackwell Publishing Ltd.; 2009:135–56.

1 › Ask the woman to empty her bladder

Ask the woman to empty her bladder, then carefully help her onto the procedure table and into the dorsal lithotomy position.

2 › Wash hands and put on protective barriers

Wash hands and put on appropriate barriers, including clean gloves.

3 › Perform a bimanual examination

Perform a bimanual examination to confirm or update findings, if an earlier assessment was done; the provider should have an accurate assessment of the uterine size and position before performing a uterine evacuation.

4 › Place the speculum

Ensure adequate visualization of the cervix.

5 › Perform cervical antiseptic preparation

Wipe the cervix with a non-alcoholic antiseptic solution, starting at the cervical os with each new sponge and spiralling outward until the os has been completely covered by antiseptic.

6 › Perform paracervical block (or proceed to Step 7)

See Section 2.3, p.27.

7 › Dilate the cervix

Dilatation is not needed when the cervix allows a cannula of appropriate size to fit snugly through the cervical os. Cervical dilatation is an essential step if the cervix is closed or insufficiently dilated. Women with incomplete abortion often already have an adequately dilated cervix.

The technique of cervical dilatation is as follows:

- carefully examine the position of the uterus and cervix and place the tenaculum on either the anterior or posterior cervical lip. With the tenaculum in place, apply continuous traction to straighten the cervical canal;

- use the smallest dilator (or a plastic os finder, if needed and available) to initially find the cervical canal;

- dilate gently, never using force, applying the no-touch technique with successive mechanical dilators, while stabilizing the cervix with gentle traction on the cervical tenaculum.

NOTE

The safety of the dilatation procedure is dependent upon adequate visibility of the cervix, gentle technique and knowledge of the uterine position. If dilatation is difficult, it is best not to force the dilator. Instead, change the angle or path to identify the cervical canal, or repeat the bimanual examination to verify the uterine position. Sometimes, changing the speculum to one with a shorter blade can provide more room and flexibility to straighten out the cervical angle. Finally, if dilatation is particularly difficult, consider administering misoprostol and delaying the procedure approximately 3 hours, or asking for assistance from a colleague, if available.

8 Insert the cannula

When appropriate cervical dilatation is achieved, insert the cannula just past the internal cervical os and into the uterine cavity while gently applying traction to the cervix.

Do not insert the cannula forcefully, to avoid trauma to the cervix or uterus.

- Stop the procedure if signs of uterine perforation occur.

IMPORTANT

It is important to use a cannula size that is appropriate to the size of the uterus and the dilatation of the cervix. Using a cannula that is too small is inefficient and may result in incomplete abortion, retained pregnancy tissue or loss of suction.

Selecting the cannula size for aspiration abortion

Uterine size (weeks since LMP*)	Suggested cannula size (mm)
4–6	4–7
7–9	5–10
9–12	8–12
12–14	10–14

*LMP: last menstrual period.

9 Aspirate the uterine contents

Attach the prepared aspirator or vacuum connection to the cannula, holding the tenaculum and the end of the cannula in one hand and the aspirator or vacuum connection in the other hand.

- Initiate the suction when the cannula tip is in mid-uterus; as the uterus contracts, the uterine walls will feel firmer and the fundus will descend.

- Evacuate the contents of the uterus by gently and slowly rotating the cannula 180° in each direction. Blood and tissue will be visible through the cannula. Do not withdraw the opening of the cannula beyond the cervical os, or suction will be lost.

- If the MVA aspirator becomes full, detach the aspirator from the cannula, leaving the cannula in the uterus, empty the aspirator into a appropriate container, and re-establish the vacuum. Repeat this procedure until the uterus is empty.

> **IMPORTANT**
>
> - The following signs indicate that the uterus is empty:
>   - red or pink foam appears and no more tissue is seen passing through the cannula;
>   - a gritty sensation is felt as the cannula passes along the surface of the evacuated uterus;
>   - the uterus contracts around the cannula;
>   - the woman feels intensified cramping or pain, indicating that the uterus is contracting.

- When the procedure is complete, remove the cannula and cervical tenaculum, wipe the cervix with a clean swab and assess the amount of uterine or cervical bleeding.

10 Inspect the tissue

Inspection of the POC is important, to ensure a complete abortion. To inspect the tissue, empty the uterine aspirate into an appropriate container (do not push aspirated contents through the cannula, as it will become contaminated).

Look for:

- the quantity and presence of POC: villi, decidua and sac/membranes in appropriate quantities based on gestational age; after 9 weeks' gestation, fetal parts are visible;
- the presence of grape-like hydropic villi, which suggest a molar pregnancy.

If the visual inspection is inconclusive, the tissue should be strained, placed in a transparent container, immersed in water or vinegar, and viewed with light from beneath. If indicated for abnormal findings, the tissue specimen may also be sent to a pathology laboratory.

- If no POC are visible, less tissue than expected was removed from the uterus, or the tissue sample is inconclusive, this may indicate:
  - incomplete abortion: the uterine cavity still contains POC, even if it appeared to be empty at the end of the procedure;
  - a spontaneous abortion that completed prior to the procedure;
  - a failed abortion: all POC remain within the uterine cavity;
  - ectopic pregnancy: when no villi are seen, ectopic pregnancy is a possibility and should be investigated;
  - anatomical anomaly: in a bicornuate or septate uterus, the cannula may have been inserted into the side of the uterus that did not contain the pregnancy.
- If it is not absolutely clear that sac/membranes and villi are present on tissue evaluation, then assume none are present and attempt re-aspiration and/or evaluate for ectopic pregnancy.

11 › Perform any concurrent procedures

When the aspiration procedure is complete, proceed with any concurrent procedures to be conducted, such as IUD insertion, tubal ligation or repairing a cervical laceration, as necessary.

12 › Recovery and discharge from the facility

- Reassure the woman that the procedure is finished and that she is no longer pregnant.
- Offer to address any emotional needs the woman might have immediately following her abortion.
- Monitor her for any complications and provide management as needed.
- She may leave the facility when she is stable and meets the criteria for discharge.
- Ensure that the woman has all necessary information and medications prior to leaving the facility.
- Document all outcomes of the treatment, including any adverse events.

Surgical abortion: >12–14 weeks of pregnancy

Clinical considerations

- The procedure for surgical abortion is called dilatation and evacuation (D&E).
- Cervical preparation with osmotic dilators or pharmacological agents is recommended prior to all D&E procedures.

Prior to the start of the procedure

- Perform cervical preparation (Refer to Surgical abortion: cervical preparation, Section 2.7).
- Provide antibiotic prophylaxis (Refer to Surgical abortion: ≤12–14 weeks, Section 2.9).
- Confirm that the woman has received her pain medications at the appropriate time.
- Ensure that all necessary equipment is gathered and available for use.

Surgical abortion
>12–14 weeks of pregnancy

1	Ask the woman to empty her bladder
2	Wash hands and put on protective barriers
3	Perform a bimanual examination
4	Place the speculum
5	Perform cervical antiseptic preparation
6	Perform paracervical block
7	Assess cervical dilatation
8	Perform amniotomy and aspirate amniotic fluid
9	Evacuate the uterus
10	Inspect the tissue
11	Perform any concurrent procedures
12	Recovery and discharge from the facility

THE "NO-TOUCH" TECHNIQUE

Follow the no-touch technique (see box on p.44) throughout the procedure.

1 › Ask the woman to empty her bladder

Ask the woman to empty her bladder, then carefully help her onto the procedure table and into the dorsal lithotomy position.

2 › Wash hands and put on protective barriers

Wash hands and put on appropriate barriers, including clean gloves.

3 › Perform a bimanual examination

Perform a bimanual examination to confirm or update findings, if an earlier assessment was done; the provider should have an accurate assessment of the uterine size and position before performing a uterine evacuation.

- If osmotic dilators were used, they should be removed from the cervix, either manually during the bimanual examination or with ring forceps after placement of the speculum. The number removed should equal the number that was placed.

4 › Place the speculum

Ensure adequate visualization of the cervix.

5 › Perform cervical antiseptic preparation

Wipe the cervix with a non-alcoholic antiseptic solution, starting at the cervical os with each new sponge and spiralling outward until the os has been completely covered by antiseptic.

6 Perform paracervical block (or proceed to Step 7)

See Section 2.3, p.27.

7 Assess cervical dilatation

Place traction on the tenaculum to bring the cervix down into the vagina. Check the adequacy of dilatation by attempting to pass a large dilator, a large-gauge cannula (12–16 mm) or Bierer forceps through the cervix. If such an instrument cannot be passed, more cervical dilatation is needed, with repeat cervical preparation or mechanical dilatation.

> **IMPORTANT**
>
> Surgical abortions should only occur if the cervix is adequately dilated. This is particularly important for abortions performed beyond 14 weeks' gestation.

8 Perform amniotomy and aspirate amniotic fluid

Insert a 14 mm cannula attached to an aspirator if using MVA, or a 14–16 mm cannula if using EVA, through the cervix into the uterine cavity, and aspirate the amniotic fluid.

- The appropriate-sized cannula (in millimetres) is generally equivalent to, or 1–2 mm less than, the gestation in weeks. For gestations greater than 16 weeks, the largest available cannula should be used (14–16 mm, depending on the tubing and cannulae available).

- Perform the suction as would be done for a first-trimester aspiration abortion, rotating the cannula during the suction to aspirate the amniotic fluid. If the cannula glides very easily back and forth through the uterus, the aperture may be blocked. In this case, remove the cannula from the uterus and clean as necessary, being careful to maintain the no-touch technique. When nothing more can be suctioned, usually after 1 or 2 minutes, remove the cannula from the uterus.

9 Evacuate the uterus

- Wherever possible, complete the evacuation from the lowest section of the uterine cavity.
- Avoid probing deeply into the uterus, particularly with instruments in the horizontal position.
- Avoid reaching high into the uterus, where the perforation risk is greater. Instead, reinsert the cannula just inside the os and use suction to bring tissue down from the fundus to the internal os.
- Stop the procedure if signs of uterine perforation occur.
- Ultrasonography may be helpful to locate fetal parts if identification is otherwise difficult. In the unlikely event that the fetal parts cannot be readily removed for any reason, consider administering a uterotonic agent, such as one of the following:
  - 400–600 µg misoprostol sublingually, orally or buccally;
  - 0.2 mg methergine orally or IM;
  - high-dose oxytocin 20 units in 500 mL normal saline or Ringer's lactate solution, run at 30 drops per minute;
  - then, reassess after 3–4 hours and repeat the uterine evacuation procedure.

10 Inspect the tissue

After the evacuation procedure, the pregnancy tissue should be evaluated to ensure complete abortion. All the following components of the pregnancy must be identified:

- four extremities;
- thorax/spine;
- calvarium;
- placenta.

If the tissue inspection indicates that the abortion may not be complete, re-evacuate the uterus or use ultrasonography to confirm complete evacuation.

11 Perform any concurrent procedures

When the aspiration procedure is complete, proceed with any concurrent procedures to be conducted such as IUD insertion or tubal ligation as requested or repairing a cervical laceration as necessary.

12 Recovery and discharge from the facility

- Reassure the woman that the procedure is finished and that she is no longer pregnant.
- Offer to address any emotional needs the woman might have immediately following her procedure.
- Monitor her for any complications and provide management as needed.
- She may leave the facility when she is stable and meets the criteria for discharge.
- Ensure that the woman has all necessary information and medications prior to leaving the facility.
- Document all outcomes of the treatment, including any adverse events.

SECTION 3

POST-ABORTION

- Prior to discharge from the health-care facility
- Additional follow-up with a health-care provider
- Post-abortion contraception
- Assessing and managing complications

OBJECTIVES

- Provide contraceptive information and offer contraceptive counselling and methods.
- Assess any other sexual and reproductive health needs that may require additional care.
- Address any immediate complications of abortion.

3.1 Prior to discharge from the health-care facility

- Provide clear oral and written discharge instructions, including:
  - sexual intercourse, douching or placing anything in the vagina should occur only after heavy bleeding stops;
  - vaginal bleeding for 2 weeks after completed surgical or medical abortion is normal. Women experience light bleeding or spotting following surgical abortion, heavier bleeding occurs with medical abortion and generally lasts for 9 days on average, but can last up to 45 days in rare cases;
  - the woman should return to the hospital or clinic if she experiences:
    - increased intensity of cramping or abdominal pain;
    - heavy vaginal bleeding;
    - fever.
- Review the risk of becoming pregnant again before her next menses, and the possible return to fertility within 2 weeks following abortion.
- Provide contraceptive information and offer contraceptive counselling to women who desire it:
  - assist her in choosing the most appropriate contraceptive method to meet her needs should she desire it;
  - provide the chosen contraceptive method (or refer her if her chosen method is not available). Ensure she knows how her selected method works, when to start it and how she can obtain future supplies.
- Provide iron tablets for anaemia, if needed.
- Provide any pain medications, if needed.
- Provide emotional support, if needed.
- Refer to other services as determined by assessment of her needs, such as STI/HIV counselling and testing, abuse support services, psychological or social services, or other physician specialists.

Additional follow-up with a health-care provider

3.2

- A routine follow-up visit is recommended only in the case of medical abortion using misoprostol alone, to assess abortion completion.

- Routine follow-up is not necessary following an uncomplicated surgical or medical abortion using mifepristone and misoprostol; however, women may be offered an optional follow-up visit 7–14 days after their procedure to provide further contraceptive counselling and methods or, further emotional support, or to address any medical concerns.

- At the follow-up appointment:
  - assess the woman's recovery and confirm completion of the abortion;
  - review any available medical records and referral documents;
  - ask about any symptoms she has experienced since the procedure;
  - perform a focused physical examination in response to any complaints;
  - assess the woman's fertility goals and need for contraceptive services:
    - if no method was started prior to discharge from the facility, provide information and offer counselling and the appropriate contraceptive method, if desired by the woman;
    - if a contraceptive method was already started:
      - assess the method used, satisfaction or concerns;
      - if she is satisfied, resupply as needed;
      - if she is not satisfied, help her select another method that will meet her needs.

- Refer to other services, as determined by assessment of her needs for additional sexual and reproductive health services, and facilitate any necessary referrals.

3.3 Post-abortion contraception*

Generally, almost all methods of contraception can be initiated immediately following a surgical or medical abortion. Immediate start of contraception after surgical abortion refers to the same day as the procedure, and for medical abortion refers to the day the first pill of a medical abortion regimen is taken. As with the initiation of any method of contraception, the woman's medical eligibility for a method should be verified.

Post-abortion medical eligibility recommendations for hormonal contraceptives, intrauterine devices and barrier contraceptive methods

POST-ABORTION CONDITION	FIRST TRIMESTER	SECOND TRIMESTER	IMMEDIATE POST-SEPTIC ABORTION
COC	1	1	1
CIC	1	1	1
Patch & vaginal ring	1	1	1
POP	1	1	1
DMPA, NET-EN	1	1	1
LNG/ETG implants	1	1	1
Copper-bearing IUD	1	2	4
LNG-releasing IUD	1	2	4
Condom	1	1	1
Spermicide	1	1	1
Diaphragm	1	1	1

CIC, combined injectable contraceptive; COC, combined oral contraceptive; DMPA/NET-EN, progestogen-only injectables: depot medroxyprogesterone acetate/norethisterone enantate; IUD, intrauterine device; LNG/ETG, progestogen-only implants: levenorgestrel/etonorgestrel; POP, progesterone-only pill.

Definition of categories
- **1:** a condition for which there is no restriction for the use of the contraceptive method.
- **2:** a condition where the advantages of using the method generally outweigh the theoretical or proven risks.
- **3:** a condition where the theoretical or proven risks usually outweigh the advantages of using the method.
- **4:** a condition that represents an unacceptable health risk if the contraceptive method is used.

*Based on Medical eligibility criteria for contraceptive use, 4th ed. Geneva: World Health Organization; 2009.

Post-abortion medical eligibility recommendations for female surgical sterilization

POST-ABORTION CONDITION	FEMALE SURGICAL STERILIZATION
Uncomplicated	A
Post-abortal sepsis or fever	D
Severe post-abortal haemorrhage	D
Severe trauma to the genital tract; cervical or vaginal tear at the time of abortion	D
Uterine perforation	S
Acute haematometra	D

Definition of categories

- **A = (accept):** there is no medical reason to deny sterilization to a person with this condition.
- **C = (caution):** the procedure is normally conducted in a routine setting, but with extra preparation and precautions.
- **D = (delay):** the procedure is delayed until the condition is evaluated and/or corrected; alternative temporary methods of contraception should be provided.
- **S = (special):** the procedure should be undertaken in a setting with an experienced surgeon and staff, and equipment is needed to provide general anaesthesia and other back-up medical support. For these conditions, the capacity to decide on the most appropriate procedure and anaesthesia regimen is also needed. Alternative temporary methods of contraception should be provided, if referral is required or there is otherwise any delay.

Contraceptive methods and medical eligibility after abortion

- **Hormonal methods (including pills, injections, implants, the patch and vaginal ring)** may be started immediately after any abortion, including septic abortion.

- **IUDs** may be inserted immediately after first- or second-trimester abortion; however, the expulsion risk is slightly higher following second-trimester abortions than following first-trimester abortions. IUDs may be inserted after a medical abortion has been deemed complete.

> **IMPORTANT**
>
> An IUD should not be inserted immediately after septic abortion.

- **Condom** use may start with the first act of sexual intercourse after abortion, including septic abortion.

- **Diaphragm or cervical cap** use may start with the first act of sexual intercourse after abortion, including septic abortion. Use should be postponed for 6 weeks following abortion beyond 14 weeks' gestation.

- **Fertility-awareness-based methods** should be delayed until regular menstrual cycles return.

- **Female surgical sterilization** can be performed immediately after uncomplicated abortions. However, it should be delayed if abortion is complicated with infection, severe haemorrhage, trauma or acute haematometra.

- **Vasectomy** can be performed at any time.

- **Emergency contraception:** women may use emergency contraceptive pills or an IUD within 5 days (120 hours) of an act of unprotected sexual intercourse, to decrease pregnancy risk.

- **Withdrawal** use may start with the first act of sexual intercourse, after abortion, including septic abortion.

Assessing and managing abortion complications 3.4

Potentially life-threatening complications are rare following safe abortion, but complications may still occur, even when taking all the necessary precautions.

When abortions are obtained from unsafe providers or locations, complications are much more common. Some women seeking subsequent care may be seriously ill and need immediate emergency attention for life-threatening conditions.

Some methods of unsafe abortion may also lead to complications related to the method used, such as ingestion of poison, toxic substances or medications, insertion of a foreign body in the anus, vagina or cervix, or abdominal trauma. Treatment of complications in these women should include treatment of any such systemic or physical injuries, in addition to any of the abortion-related complications.

Ongoing pregnancy

- Women with continuing signs of pregnancy or clinical signs of failed abortion should be offered a uterine evacuation in a timely fashion.

Incomplete abortion

Common symptoms of incomplete abortion include vaginal bleeding and abdominal pain. It should also be suspected if, upon inspection, the POC aspirated during surgical abortion is not compatible with the estimated duration of pregnancy.

- Incomplete abortion following spontaneous or induced abortion may be managed similarly.

- Clinically stable patients have the following three options:
  - expectant management;
  - vacuum aspiration: (for uterine size of up to 14 weeks' gestation);
  - management with misoprostol (for uterine size of up to 13 weeks' gestation).

- The decision should be based upon the clinical condition of the woman and her preferences for treatment.

Recommended regimen for management of incomplete abortion with misoprostol

DOSE (µg)	ROUTE
600 µg	Oral
400 µg	Sublingual
400–800 µg	Vaginal; may be used if vaginal bleeding is minimal

Comparison of management options for missed and incomplete abortions

METHOD	POTENTIAL ADVANTAGES	POTENTIAL DISADVANTAGES	EFFICACY (%) Missed	EFFICACY (%) Incomplete
Expectant management[a]	- May minimize visits - Avoids side-effects and complications of other methods - Avoids intrauterine instrumentation	- Unpredictable time frame - May still require follow-up aspiration if not successful	16–75	82–100
Misoprostol alone	- Avoids intrauterine instrumentation	- May cause more bleeding and need for follow-up than aspiration - Short-term side-effects from misoprostol	77–89	61–100
Aspiration	- Quick resolution	- Surgical procedure	96–100	96–100

[a] The efficacy of expectant management increases with increasing interval before intervention.

Source: adapted from Goodman S, Wolfe M and the TEACH Trainers Collaborative Working Group. Early abortion training workbook, 3rd ed. San Francisco: UCSF Bixby Center for Reproductive Health Research and Policy; 2007, with permission.

Assessing and managing abortion complications

3.4

Potentially life-threatening complications are rare following safe abortion, but complications may still occur, even when taking all the necessary precautions.

When abortions are obtained from unsafe providers or locations, complications are much more common. Some women seeking subsequent care may be seriously ill and need immediate emergency attention for life-threatening conditions.

Some methods of unsafe abortion may also lead to complications related to the method used, such as ingestion of poison, toxic substances or medications, insertion of a foreign body in the anus, vagina or cervix, or abdominal trauma. Treatment of complications in these women should include treatment of any such systemic or physical injuries, in addition to any of the abortion-related complications.

Ongoing pregnancy

- Women with continuing signs of pregnancy or clinical signs of failed abortion should be offered a uterine evacuation in a timely fashion.

Incomplete abortion

Common symptoms of incomplete abortion include vaginal bleeding and abdominal pain. It should also be suspected if, upon inspection, the POC aspirated during surgical abortion is not compatible with the estimated duration of pregnancy.

- Incomplete abortion following spontaneous or induced abortion may be managed similarly.

- Clinically stable patients have the following three options:
  - expectant management;
  - vacuum aspiration: (for uterine size of up to 14 weeks' gestation);
  - management with misoprostol (for uterine size of up to 13 weeks' gestation).

- The decision should be based upon the clinical condition of the woman and her preferences for treatment.

Recommended regimen for management of incomplete abortion with misoprostol

DOSE (µg)	ROUTE
600 µg	Oral
400 µg	Sublingual
400–800 µg	Vaginal; may be used if vaginal bleeding is minimal

Comparison of management options for missed and incomplete abortions

METHOD	POTENTIAL ADVANTAGES	POTENTIAL DISADVANTAGES	EFFICACY (%) Missed	EFFICACY (%) Incomplete
Expectant management[a]	▪ May minimize visits ▪ Avoids side-effects and complications of other methods ▪ Avoids intrauterine instrumentation	▪ Unpredictable time frame ▪ May still require follow-up aspiration if not successful	16–75	82–100
Misoprostol alone	▪ Avoids intrauterine instrumentation	▪ May cause more bleeding and need for follow-up than aspiration ▪ Short-term side-effects from misoprostol	77–89	61–100
Aspiration	▪ Quick resolution	▪ Surgical procedure	96–100	96–100

[a] The efficacy of expectant management increases with increasing interval before intervention.

Source: adapted from Goodman S, Wolfe M and the TEACH Trainers Collaborative Working Group. Early abortion training workbook, 3rd ed. San Francisco: UCSF Bixby Center for Reproductive Health Research and Policy; 2007, with permission.

Haemorrhage

Haemorrhage can result from retained POC, trauma or damage to the cervix, coagulopathy or, rarely, uterine perforation or uterine rupture.

- Appropriate treatment for haemorrhage depends on its cause and severity, and includes:
    - re-evacuation of the uterus;
    - administration of uterotonic drugs;
    - blood transfusion;
    - replacement of clotting factors;
    - laparoscopy;
    - exploratory laparotomy.
- Every service-delivery site must be able to stabilize and treat or refer women with haemorrhage immediately.

Infection

- Common signs and symptoms of infection include:
    - fever or chills;
    - foul-smelling vaginal or cervical discharge;
    - abdominal or pelvic pain;
    - prolonged vaginal bleeding or spotting;
    - uterine tenderness;
    - an elevated white blood cell count.
- Women with infection require antibiotics for treatment.
- If retained POC are suspected to be a cause for infection, re-evacuate the uterus.
- Women with severe infections may require hospitalization.

Uterine perforation

- Uterine perforation usually goes undetected and resolves without the need for intervention.
- When available and necessary, laparoscopy is the investigative method of choice.
- If the woman's status or findings during laparoscopy suggest damage to the bowel, blood vessels or other structures, a laparotomy to repair any damage may be needed.

Anaesthesia-related complications

- Where general anaesthesia is used, staff must be skilled in the management of seizures and cardiorespiratory resuscitation.
- Narcotic-reversal agents should always be readily available in settings where narcotics are used.

Complications may occur that are not specific to the abortion procedure

These include:

- anaphylaxis;
- asthmatic reactions.

These complications should be treated as they would be following any other procedure.

Notes: